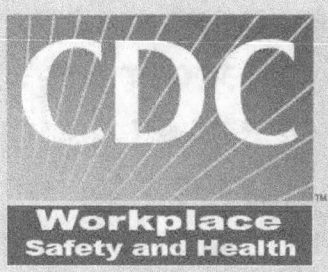

Evaluation of Exposure to Radon Progeny During Closure of Inactive Uranium Mines – Colorado

Robert D. Daniels, PhD, CHP
David C. Sylvain, MS, CIH

Health Hazard Evaluation Report
HETA 2011-0090-3161
July 2012

DEPARTMENT OF HEALTH AND HUMAN SERVICES
Centers for Disease Control and Prevention

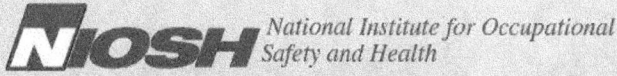 National Institute for Occupational Safety and Health

The employer shall post a copy of this report for a period of 30 calendar days at or near the workplace(s) of affected employees. The employer shall take steps to insure that the posted determinations are not altered, defaced, or covered by other material during such period. [37 FR 23640, November 7, 1972, as amended at 45 FR 2653, January 14, 1980].

CONTENTS

ABBREVIATIONS

ACGIH®	American Conference of Governmental Industrial Hygienists
ALARA	As low as reasonably achievable
ALI	Annual limit on intake
Bq	Becquerel
CFR	Code of Federal Regulations
CI	Confidence interval
Ci	Curie
CWLM	Continuous working level monitor
DCF	Dose conversion factor
DOE	Department of Energy
EEC	Equilibrium equivalent concentration
EPA	Environmental Protection Agency
F_{eq}	Equilibrium factor
Gy	Gray
h^{-1}	Per hour
HHE	Health hazard evaluation
ICRP	International Commission on Radiological Protection
J	Joules
L^{-1}	Per liter
m^{-3}	Per cubic meter
MeV	Mega electron volt (10^6 eV)
MSHA	Mine Safety and Health Administration
NAICS	North American Industry Classification System
NCRP	National Council on Radiation Protection and Measurements
NIOSH	National Institute for Occupational Safety and Health
NRC	Nuclear Regulatory Commission
OEL	Occupational Exposure Limit
OSHA	Occupational Safety and Health Administration
PAEC	Potential alpha energy concentration
PEL	Permissible exposure limit
PPE	Personal protective equipment
REL	Recommended exposure limit
Sv	Sievert
TLV®	Threshold limit value
UNSCEAR	United Nations Scientific Committee on the Effects of Atomic Radiation
WL	Working level
WLM^{-1}	Per working level month
WLM	Working level month
y^{-1}	Per year

HIGHLIGHTS OF THE NIOSH HEALTH HAZARD EVALUATION

The National Institute for Occupational Safety and Health (NIOSH) received a request for a health hazard evaluation at abandoned uranium mines in several western states. Managers of a federal agency requested assistance in evaluating employee exposures to radon while constructing mine closures.

What NIOSH Did

- We evaluated mines in Colorado and Utah in September 2011.
- We measured radon levels at several mine openings.
- We measured gamma radiation dose rates on the surface of an abandoned ore and waste rock pile.
- We observed the construction of a stone and mortar closure.
- We reviewed past exposure data collected by the state inactive mine reclamation program in Colorado.

What NIOSH Found

- Workplace radon concentrations were affected by changing environmental conditions.
- The potential for workplace exposures to radon was low. Controls were needed in some instances to keep exposures as low as reasonably achievable.
- Gamma radiation was measureable at the surface of the waste rock pile.

What Managers Can Do

- Inform employees about radiation hazards in the workplace.
- Adopt reference levels that would prompt the use of control measures.
- Improve environmental monitoring that is done pre-bid. This will allow for more accurate estimates of potential exposures.
- Use fans to provide dilution ventilation at mine openings.
- Construct temporary radon barriers at mine openings.
- Plan work before arriving at the worksite. This will minimize the amount of time spent working near mine openings.
- Provide respiratory protection to employees. Respirators can be used to control exposures when engineering and administrative controls are not sufficient.

What Employees Can Do

- Learn about potential exposures and hazards at mine sites.
- Use temporary barriers, dilution ventilation, and good work practices to minimize your exposure to radiation hazards.

HIGHLIGHTS OF THE NIOSH HEALTH HAZARD EVALUATION (CONTINUED)

- Plan work before arriving at the worksite so you spend less time working near mine openings.
- Participate in training offered by your employer.
- Use the appropriate personal protective equipment when recommended.

SUMMARY

NIOSH evaluated employee exposures to radon progeny and gamma radiation during the construction of mine closures. We found that exposures were generally low, but were influenced by environmental conditions. NIOSH measurements were similar to those obtained by the state inactive mine reclamation program. Recommendations for the use of simple engineering controls and respiratory protection are made in the report to keep exposures ALARA.

In June 2011, NIOSH received an HHE request from managers of a federal agency in Colorado. NIOSH was asked to evaluate employees' exposure to ionizing radiation hazards during construction of various types of closures at abandoned uranium mines. The primary health concern at these sites involved inhalation of naturally occurring short-lived radon progeny (i.e., polonium-218, lead-214, bismuth-214, and polonium-214) at mine entrances (adits). Also of concern, but to a lesser extent, was exposure to gamma radiation emitted from mine waste and nearby geological formations.

On September 12–15, 2011, we visited several abandoned mines on Wedding Bell Mountain in southwest Colorado and the Vanadium Queen mine in Utah. We observed the construction of a native stone and mortar closure on Wedding Bell Mountain. We also conducted continuous monitoring of radon progeny at several mine openings at Wedding Bell Mountain and at the Vanadium Queen mine. We reviewed the state inactive mine reclamation program's pre-bid radon monitoring protocol.

Monitoring results and onsite observations suggest that employee exposures to radon during mine closure activities are generally low. However, radon concentrations at mine openings are greatly affected by changing environmental conditions such as wind velocity, moisture, and barometric pressure. Results of NIOSH exposure monitoring did not exceed the average pre-bid PAEC values obtained during previous monitoring by state inactive mine reclamation program staff. Nevertheless, PAEC results from the CWLMs varied widely over the sampling period because of constant fluctuations in ventilation patterns. Given this variability, it is unlikely that short-term sampling, as conducted by state inactive mine reclamation program staff, is sufficient to derive long-term average concentrations that form the basis of protective actions.

Control measures are needed in some instances to keep exposures ALARA. Gamma radiation is likely to be measureable at the surface of waste rock piles near mine adits. Occupancy to these areas should be limited to minimize exposures to radon. The use of simple engineering controls (e.g., barriers, ventilation), along with the use of respiratory protection when needed, are recommended to keep radon exposures ALARA.

Keywords: NAICS 924120 (Administration of Conservation Programs), radon, radon progeny, gamma radiation, inactive mine reclamation, uranium mines

INTRODUCTION

In June 2011, NIOSH received an HHE request from the managers of a federal agency. NIOSH was asked to evaluate employee exposure to ionizing radiation hazards during construction of various types of closures at abandoned uranium mines on federal land. The primary health concern at these sites involves inhalation of naturally occurring short-lived radon progeny (i.e., polonium-218, lead-214, bismuth-214, and polonium-214) at mine entrances (adits), and, to a lesser extent, exposure to gamma radiation emitted from mine waste and geological formations. NIOSH visited several mines on Wedding Bell Mountain in southwest Colorado on September 12–13, 2011, and the Vanadium Queen mine in Utah on September 14, 2011. This report summarizes the findings of the site visit and our assessment of the radiological hazards at the mines.

Background

Uranium exploration, mining, and ore processing in the United States have resulted in a number of abandoned sites that present significant occupational and environmental hazards. Efforts are ongoing to mitigate these hazards. One such effort is the safe closure of abandoned underground uranium mines, which entails installation of permanent barriers at mine openings to prevent the public from entering the mines. The mines are principally located in remote areas of the Four Corners region of Colorado, Arizona, New Mexico, and Utah. Mine closure activities present numerous physical hazards that are exacerbated by the rugged terrain and isolation at mine locations. Primary hazards include (1) construction hazards associated with trenching, excavation, and heavy equipment operations; (2) environmental hazards such as inclement weather, mountainous terrain (e g , falling rock, elevated work), and wildlife; and (3) hazards associated with isolation from communications, utilities, emergency response, and medical services.

Additionally, employees are exposed to ionizing radiation from technologically enhanced naturally occurring radioactive material, comprised of primordial naturally-occurring radioactive elements, such as radium, uranium, and thorium and their radioactive decay products that have been concentrated or made environmentally accessible during mining activities. In general, radiation-related occupational hazards at mine closure sites are due to inhalation of radon gas and its short-lived decay products that emanate from mine openings and, to a lesser extent, exposure to elevated levels of gamma radiation where radium is present.

INTRODUCTION (CONTINUED)

Abandoned mines that are subject to closure no longer have operational ventilation systems; therefore, mine atmospheres may contain radon progeny in much higher concentrations than are found in operating mines. Although airborne radioactivity is likely to be less at mine openings because of fresh air mixing, employees working near the adits and other openings could be exposed to significant levels of contaminated air from outcasting (exhaling) mine atmospheres. For this reason, radon hazards to employees supporting mine reclamation were evaluated in this HHE. These employees do not make mine entries; therefore, this evaluation did not consider the risk to personnel (employees or the public) who enter and occupy mine spaces.

ASSESSMENT

Review of Prior State Radiation Monitoring

As an integral part of the Wedding Bell Mine Safety Closure Project, staff from the state inactive mine reclamation program measured PAEC at least twice at each mine opening that was identified on the bid schedule. The first measurement ("pre-bid" sample) was performed to gather information necessary for the development of construction specifications that are included in the contract solicitation. A second PAEC measurement was made in the presence of the contractor after the contract was awarded, but during pre-construction activities. The selected contractor is instructed to use the higher of the two (or more) samples in the planning of work activities. All measurements are compiled from data collected during 15-minute short-term samples using the Bladewerx SabreAlert2™ (Bladewerx, Rio Rancho, New Mexico).

State inactive mine reclamation program staff also conducted gamma radiation surveys using a Delta Epsilon SC-133 (Delta Epsilon Instruments, Inc., Grand Junction, Colorado) handheld portable scintillometer (gamma dose rate meter) at the Wedding Bell Mountain sites. Data on 45 survey points at various work locations at Wedding Bell Mountain were compiled for the active work under observation.

NIOSH Radiation Monitoring

We conducted continuous radon progeny monitoring at several mine openings at Wedding Bell Mountain on September 12–13,

ASSESSMENT (COINTINUED)

2011, and at the Vanadium Queen mine in southeast Utah on September 14, 2011. Although not a part of the Wedding Bell Mine Safety Closure Project, the Vanadium Queen mine was selected because of its proximity to the Fire Fly mine, which was referenced in a draft report that measured high airborne alpha radiation concentrations inside and near abandoned uranium mines [Duraski 2010]. The primary instrument used by NIOSH was a model 597-PX3 Continuous Working Level Monitor (alphaNUCLEAR, Saskatchewan, Canada), which was specifically manufactured for the Canadian uranium mining industry. Measurements were also obtained with the Bladewerx SabreAlert2, which is the current instrument used by the state inactive mine reclamation program. Each monitor was factory calibrated within 6 months of use; however, only the 597-PX3 was tested in a radon chamber. Both instruments are fully-contained, battery-powered, microprocessor-based, continuous-area monitors that incorporate an air pump, sample filter, and radioactivity counting system to calculate individual radon progeny concentrations via alpha spectral analysis. Both monitors have data logging capability and provide for short-term (acute), and long-term (chronic) WL measurements. Short-term measurements are less precise than long-term; however, shorter sampling intervals allow for quicker responses to transient airborne concentrations that are common to mine atmospheres. The monitors were placed in the work areas as close to the mine opening as possible. Smoke tubes were used to visualize air movement at the monitoring site and other workplace locations. On the basis of the observed work practices, occupancy, and ventilation patterns, continuous area monitoring was likely to overestimate worker exposures.

Gamma radiation surveys were conducted by NIOSH and state inactive mine reclamation program staff using the SC-133 handheld portable scintillometer manufactured by Delta Epsilon Instruments, Inc.

Review of Prior State Radiation Monitoring

Potential Alpha Energy Concentration

Forty-six pre-bid radon monitoring results were reported for the closure activities identified in the current bid schedule. Sample results were available for 40 adits, 4 shafts, and 2 vents. The sample distribution was highly right-skewed, with arithmetic mean, median, and 95th percentile values of 0.31 WL, 0.04 WL, and 1.5 WL. The maximum recorded PAEC value was 4.2 WL at a small vent (897 V1) that was scheduled for a polyurethane foam closure. The adit PAEC ranged from 0.005 to 1.55 WL with mean and median values of 0.24 and 0.05 WL. Twelve (30%) short-term samples exceeded 0.1 WL, of which all but one were assigned to an adit.

Gamma Radiation

Prior monitoring at the Wedding Bell Mountain sites with a handheld portable scintillometer (gamma dose rate meter) indicated dose rates ranging from 0.13 to 4.8 μSv·h^{-1} with a mean dose rate of 1.0 μSv·h^{-1} (95% CI: 0.8–1 3) from all sources including background.

NIOSH Radiation Monitoring

Potential Alpha Energy Concentration

Average PAEC values at Wedding Bell Mountain mine locations were within the range of expected values on the basis of data from the state inactive mine reclamation program pre-bid short-term samples (Table 1). The highest Wedding Bell Mountain mine progeny concentrations were observed at Adit 908A3, where transient (i.e., short-term) WL concentrations exceeded 1.0 WL during a period of rapidly changing weather conditions. During this time, long-term concentrations did not exceed 0.5 WL. In contrast, transient PAEC concentrations in excess of 10 WL were found at one of two Utah Vanadium Queen mine adits (VQ1). The highest concentrations were obtained approximately 0 5 meter above the mine floor, which was completely submerged with groundwater at the time of sampling. The other opening (VQ2) was dry, although both mine entrances were believed to be interconnected.

Table 1. PAECs from continuous monitoring

Date	Location	Pre-bid WL	597-PX3		SabreAlert2 WL	
			Avg. WL (range)*	Run hours	WL (range)*	Run hours
9-12-2011	908A5	0.007	NM†	NM	0.0003 (0.0–0.0008)	0.33
9-12-2011	907S1	NM	0.01 (0.0–0.03)	1.1	0.004 (0.0–0.012)	1.1
9-13-2011	896A12	0.0084	NM	NM	0.003 (0.0–0.010)	0.75
9-13-2011	908A3	0.989	0.25 (0.0–1.1)	5.7	0.136 (0.04–0.31)	1.0
9-14-2011	VQ1	NM	6.98 (0–14.38)	1.0	0.431 (0.003–1.265)	1.0
9-14-2011	VQ2	NM	0.91 (0.1–3.25)	2.7	0.078 (0.0–0.984)	2.7

*Values are from "short-term" or "acute" WL measurement algorithms.
†NM=not measured

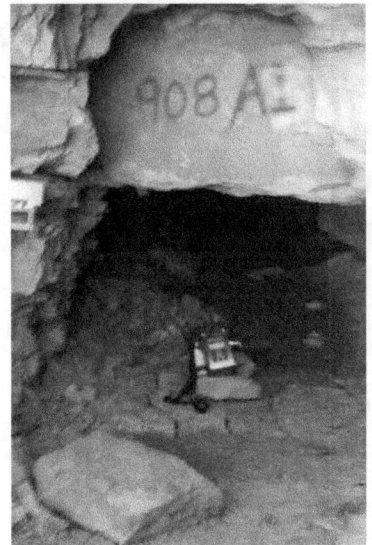

Figure 1. Wedding Bell Mountain Adit 908A3 monitoring on September 13, 2011.

Although radon gas measurements were not taken, both CWLMs calculated F_{eq} values from progeny results. These fractions typically ranged between 0.2 and 0.7; average values for the SabreAlert2 were 0 3 and for the 597-PX3 were 0.5. Although Feq values were in reasonable agreement with recommended values of 0.4 for indoor air and 0.7 for outdoors [ICRP 1993], the actual algorithms used by the CWLMs to determine F_{eq} were not made available, thus the validity of these estimates could not be determined. Differences in algorithms may partly explain measurement inconsistencies between monitor types.

Wedding Bell Mountain Adit 908A3

Continuous PAEC monitoring using both monitors was conducted at Adit 908A3 on September 13, 2011 (Table 1). This adit closure had not been initiated at the time of sampling, and the planned closure method requires the installation of a corrugated steel pipe and bat gate. The final pre-bid WL for this opening was 0.989 WL, which was taken during observed outflow.

The 597-PX3 was operated from 11:18 to 16:58 hours (5.7 hours). The SabreAlert2 was operated from 11:34 to 12:32 (about 1.0 hour). As shown in Figure 1, the 597-PX3 was placed near the side of the adit at a height of about one meter, while the SabreAlert2 monitor was placed at ground level at the center of the opening.

The weather conditions at the beginning of the sampling period were sunny and clear with a mild swirling wind. Intermittent outflow from the adit was evident by smoke tube visualization and by a pronounced variability in air temperature at the adit during the monitoring period. During the time period of approximately one hour when both monitors were operated simultaneously, the average short-term PAEC values were 0.15 WL (range: 0.05–0.24) for the 597-PX3 and 0.136 WL (range: 0.04–0.31) for the SabreAlert2.

The short-term results from both monitors were in reasonable agreement; however, results from the long-term algorithm of the 597-PX3 were consistently higher than those reported by the SabreAlert2 (Figure 2). During this period, neither monitor indicated results that exceeded pre-bid levels.

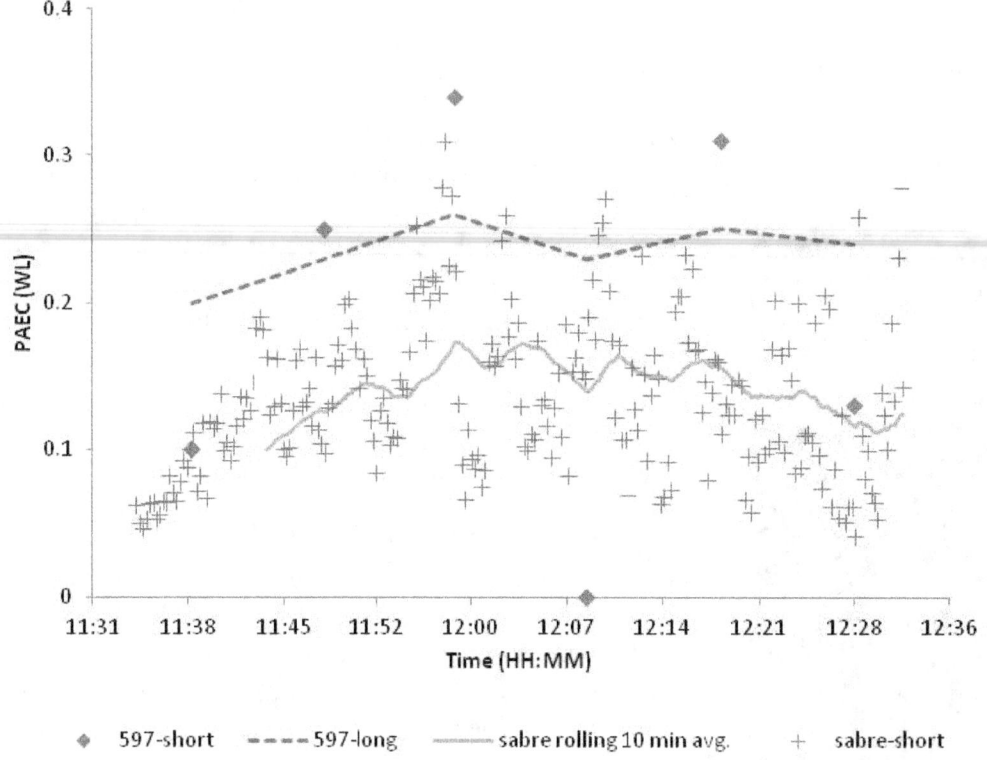

Figure 2. PAEC monitoring data for Wedding Bell Mountain Adit 908A3 on September 13, 2011.

SabreAlert2 monitoring was discontinued at approximately 12:30 hours, and the 597-PX3 was relocated to the vacated position. The change in position resulted in a slight reduction in the short-term PAEC measurements. A plastic tarp was installed at the adit as a temporary barrier at approximately 14:00 hours. During this time, the 597-PX3 was positioned about 0.5 meters from the ground (Figure 3). The barrier was hastily constructed from available materials resulting in a poor seal; nevertheless, a noticeable reduction in the PAEC was evident immediately following installation (Figure 4). The barrier remained in place throughout the rest of the monitoring period.

RESULTS
(CONTINUED)

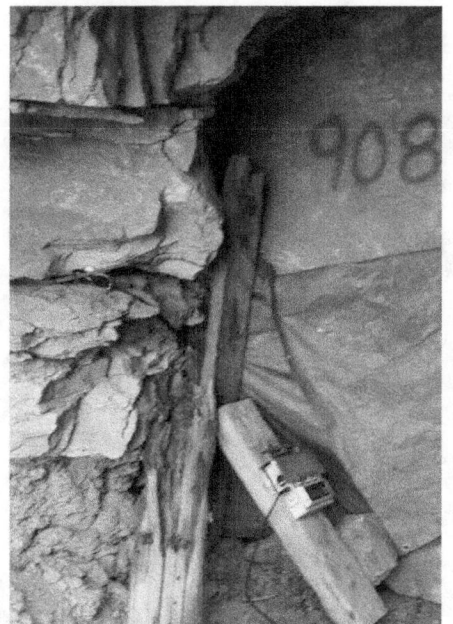

Figure 3. Temporary barrier installed at Wedding Bell Mountain Adit 908A3.

A weather front was observed during the afternoon (approximately 15:30 hours) with the onset of cloudy conditions, increased wind, mild rain, and a drop in barometric pressure. A marked increase in outflow frequency and level coincided with the changing weather conditions, resulting in steadily rising PAEC levels that peaked above 1.0 WL (Figure 4). Monitoring was discontinued at about 17:00 hours.

Vanadium Queen Mine Adits

Two adits were sampled on September 14, 2011. Both adits were part of the Vanadium Queen mine in the La Sal Creek Canyon located in southeast Utah. Neither of these adits is included in the Colorado reclamation contract; therefore, no pre-bid samples had been collected by state inactive mine reclamation program staff. Adit VQ1 was approximately 1 5 meters by 1.5 meters without a closure device. The floor of the mine was covered with standing water. This groundwater continuously drained from the adit to form a small stream down the side the mountain. Based on

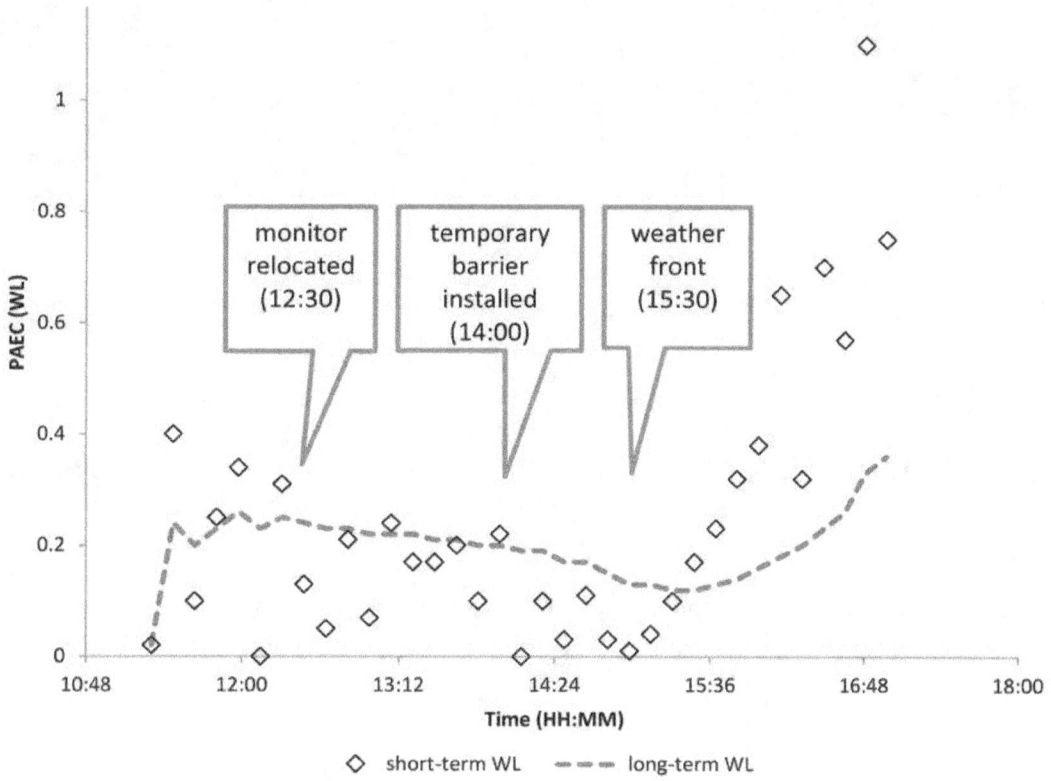

Figure 4. PAEC monitoring data for Wedding Bell Mountain Adit 908A3 on September 13, 2011, using the 597-PX3.

vegetation growth, the mine drainage pattern appeared to be long term. Adit VQ2 was approximately 100 meters from VQ1, situated along the same ridgeline of the mountain. Standing water was not present at the second adit and there was no evidence of drainage from the mine. Weather conditions were cool and cloudy with light rain throughout the entire monitoring period.

Sampling at VQ1 with the 597-PX3 started at approximately 12:00 hours on September 14, 2011. Because of the poor weather conditions and rising water levels in and around the adit, sampling was discontinued at 13:12 hours. During this short monitoring period, the average PAEC at VQ1 was nearly 7.0 WL (range 0.0–14.38), although levels steadily declined after the first 20 minutes of monitoring (Figure 5). In contrast, the average PAEC at the dry location (VQ2) was 0.91 WL (range: 0.1–3.25) (Table 1 and Figure 6).

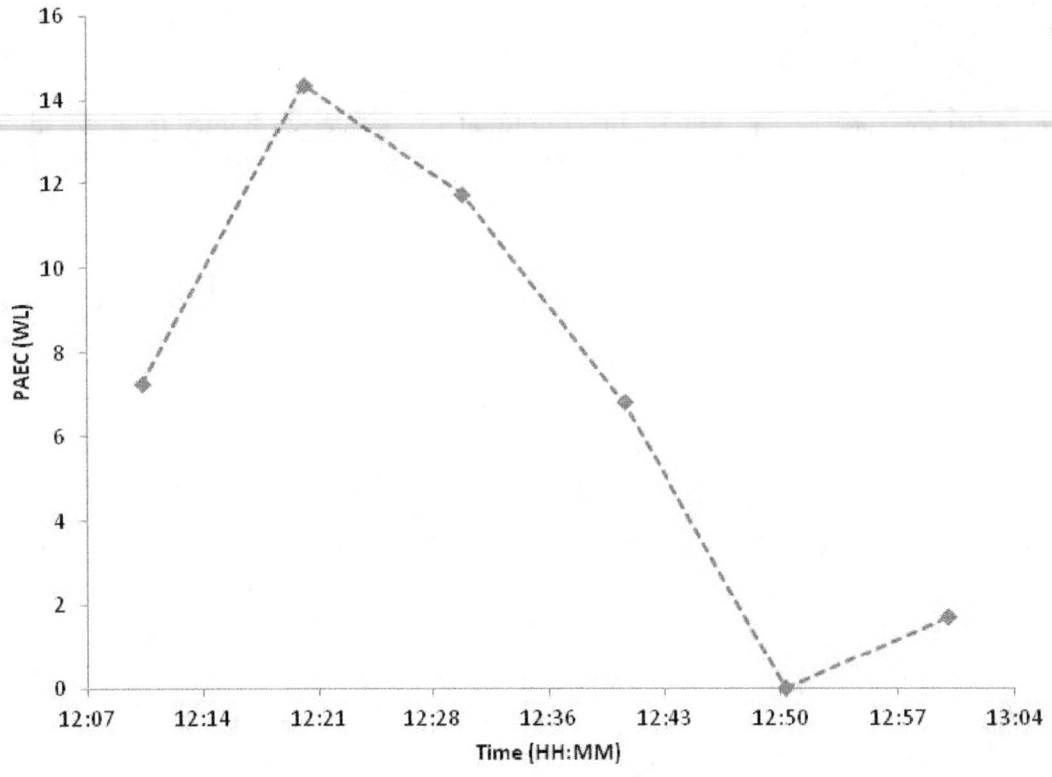

Figure 5. Continuous PAEC monitoring at VQ1 on September 14, 2011.

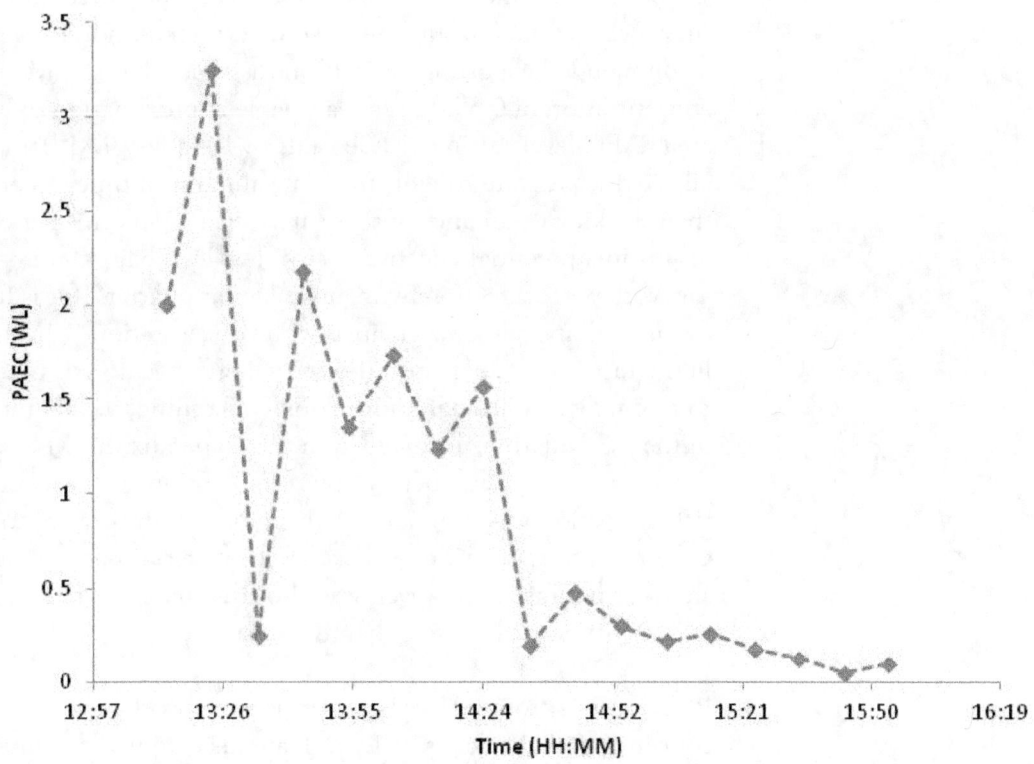

Figure 6. Continuous PAEC monitoring at VQ2 on September 14, 2011.

Gamma radiation monitoring by NIOSH investigators at the Vanadium Queen mine indicated that dose rates were typically near background levels; however, peak dose rates in excess of 10 $\mu Sv \cdot h^{-1}$ were measured on the surface of an abandoned ore and waste rock pile. The general area dose rate at about 30 centimeters from the pile surface was approximately 3.0 $\mu Sv \cdot h^{-1}$.

Discussion

Review of monitoring data from the state inactive mine reclamation program showed that the distribution of short-term sampling radon measurements was highly right skewed and suggested that few closure areas required intervention for achieving recommended exposure levels. If one assumes that the average concentration of 0 3 WL is a reasonable approximation of work area PAEC levels (using a DCF value of 10 mSv·WLM^{-1}) and that all activities require roughly the same amount of time to complete, then working occupancy of these areas over a 9-month period results in a potential effective dose of just less than 30 mSv for the work year and <10 mSv in any calendar quarter. If it is further assumed that occupancy in areas with concentrations >1WL is limited to 4 hours per shift, the annual effective dose is reduced to ~16 mSv. Additional information concerning the assumptions in these calculations is included in the Appendix. In this example, regulatory limits were met without intervention, and reasonable risk mitigation was achievable with simple administrative controls. Of course, this assertion is weakened by uncertain results from short-term samples; however, it is also true that actual closure work may consume far less time than that assumed.

PAEC results from CWLMs confirmed that work area concentrations in excess of 1.0 WL are likely to be encountered at some closure sites where standing water is present and/or outcasting mine atmospheres is common. Considerable outcasting from adits was easily identifiable by a sharp temperature difference when approaching the opening, with cooler air signifying escaping mine air. Careful attention to weather conditions, mine ventilation patterns, and standing water should alert employees to excessive radon environments and trigger protective measures.

There were differences in results observed between the 597-PX3 and SabreAlert2 CWLMs. Some differences are expected because of dissimilar design characteristics and computational algorithms. However, relatively large disparities between monitors at high concentrations emphasize the need for formal intercomparisons under controlled conditions.

Average PAEC values from NIOSH exposure monitoring did not exceed pre-bid levels from previous monitoring by state inactive mine reclamation program staff. Nevertheless, PAEC results from the CWLMs varied widely over the sampling period because of constant fluctuations in ventilation patterns caused by changing environmental conditions. Given this variability, it is unlikely that short-term sampling, as conducted by state inactive mine

DISCUSSION (CONTINUED)

reclamation program staff, is sufficient to derive long-term average concentrations that form the basis of protective actions. If CWLMs are used for work area characterizations, then sampling periods should be maximized (preferably >3 hours) or multiple short-term measurements be conducted. As an alternative to short-term sampling, long-term radon monitoring using inexpensive passive monitors (e.g., CR-39 alpha-track detectors or electrets) may provide a better characterization of potential radon hazards at mine reclamation sites. For example, pre-bid radon characterization could be accomplished with CR-39 based alpha-track radon gas detectors designed for outdoor area monitoring (e.g , Landauer® Radtrak®, Landauer, Inc., Glenwood, Illinois). The typical detection capability of these monitors is about 1.1 $kBq \cdot m^{-3} \cdot d$ (30 $pCi \cdot L^{-1} \cdot d$); therefore, an average concentration of 160 $Bq \cdot m^{-3}$ (4.3 $pCi \cdot L^{-1}$) is detectable in a 7-day sample period. Assuming 40% daughter equilibrium, continuous exposure at 160 $Bq \cdot m^{-3}$ over a working year (2,000 hours) results in about 0.2 WLM or about 2 mSv annual effective dose. Longer sample periods will increase sensitivity and further reduce uncertainties from seasonal and diurnal variations. Results from weekly or biweekly sampling would better support decisions on radiological controls included in the bid specifications for reclamation work. Moreover, as more information becomes available from long-term sampling, patterns may arise in the data that may be used in predictive models that reduce the need for additional characterization by sampling.

Gamma monitoring by state inactive mine reclamation program staff and NIOSH indicated that hazards from external exposures were small relative to radon exposures. In most instances, radiation levels were indistinguishable from background; however, elevated dose rates were found near an abandoned ore pile at one mine location. Assuming continuous occupancy (2,000 hours) in areas with dose rates ranging from 1 $\mu Sv \cdot h^{-1}$ to 5 $\mu Sv \cdot h^{-1}$ (i.e., mean and maximum levels measured by state inactive mine reclamation program staff) results in annual doses between 2 mSv and 10 mSv. Therefore, the potential dose equivalent contribution from external irradiation is generally far less than regulatory limits and appears negligible when compared to the effective dose from radon.

As a potential exception, the dose equivalent to an embryo or fetus should be kept ALARA and below 5 mSv over the gestation period. Therefore, additional controls (e.g., work restrictions) may be necessary to limit external exposures to the declared pregnant worker. In the absence of uptakes of long-lived radionuclides associated with technologically enhanced naturally occurring radioactive material, the radiation hazard to the fetus is limited to the dose equivalent from external exposures to gamma radiation. The fetal dose-equivalent from radon and short-lived radon progeny exposures is very small (about 0.1 mSv·WLM^{-1}) and is not considered a limiting factor in decisions regarding radon exposures [Richardson et al. 1991; Kendall and Smith 2002; Kendall et al. 2009].

Radiological Controls

The fundamental principles of justification and optimization are recommended for establishing appropriate radiological controls to reduce the hazard of radon exposure [ICRP 2007]. Justification explicitly refers to weighing the benefit of activity against the consequences of the exposure and judging that the net benefit is positive. Optimization of protection is achieved when radiation doses to the individual or individuals are ALARA, taking into account economic and societal factors. The optimization process involves four basic steps:

1. Evaluation of the exposure situation
2. Selection of an appropriate constraint or reference level
3. Identification of control options
4. Selection and implementation of the preferred option

In this case, the reference level (constraint) is considered as a basic level of protection and is always established (for planned exposures or existing controllable exposure situations) as some value below the applicable dose limits, which in U.S. protection systems are generally equivalent to 4 WLM·y^{-1} for radon and 50 mSv·y^{-1} for effective dose.

Selection of a Reference Level

The ICRP recommends an annual reference level of 10 mSv effective dose from radon, above which doses should be considered "occupational" and require radiological control intervention [ICRP 2007]. Assuming continuous occupancy in a work year (2,000 hours), the reference level is equivalent to the NIOSH REL of 1 WLM·y^{-1}. Additionally, the reference level can be equated to

DISCUSSION
(CONTINUED)

a continuous workshift-averaged PAEC value of 1.7×10^{-3} mJ·m^{-3} (0.083 WL) and a radon concentration of about 800 Bq·m^{-3} (22 pCi·L^{-1}) assuming 40% equilibrium (F_{eq}=0.4). This appears to be in reasonable agreement with thresholds for posting and controls specified by the major U.S. regulatory agencies [10 CFR 835; 10 CFR 20; 29 CFR 1926.53] as discussed in the Appendix. Note that the recommended reference level is based on 2,000-hour occupancy, which is not feasible for mine closure activities because of inclement weather conditions during the winter. Assuming that work is limited to a 9-month period (1,500 hours) the reference PAEC is about 2×10^{-3} mJ·m^{-3} (0.1 WL), and the radon concentration is about 1 kBq·m^{-3} (27 pCi·L^{-1} as shown in Table 2.

Table 2. Recommended radon annual reference levels*

Effective dose	Exposure	PAEC	Radon 222 concentration
10 mSv (1 rem)	3.54 J·h·m^{-3} (1 WLM·y^{-1})	2×10^{-3} mJ·m^{-3} (0.1 WL)	1kBq·m^{-3} (27 pCi·L^{-1})

*PAEC and radon 222 concentration values assume 75% occupancy in a working year (i.e., 1,500 hours).

The reference level establishes a threshold for intervention under conservative assumptions. In this case, workplace controls are considered if a worker's annual effective dose from radon exposure is likely to exceed 10 mSv if left unmitigated. Compliance with the reference level is assured by average PAEC concentrations less than 0.1 WL and yearly occupancy no more than 1,500 hours. Current estimates from occupancy records suggest that individuals involved in mine closure activities spend far less than 1,500 hours per year at the work site because of funding constraints, procurement regulations, and other work preparation activities. Reference concentration values may be adjusted upward on the basis of improved occupancy estimates and assurances that the annual effective dose goal of 10 mSv (1 WLM) is maintained.

State inactive mine reclamation program staff had established ALARA goals for mine reclamation work and have incorporated these goals into its most recent revision to mine safety procedures included in contract specifications. The state inactive mine reclamation program goals are similar to, but slightly less conservative than, the proposed reference level. The state inactive mine reclamation program goals are not to exceed 15 mSv effective dose from radon and 20 mSv dose-equivalent from external irradiation. On the basis of an assumed annual occupancy of 800 hours, a DCF of 8.6 mSv·WLM^{-1}, and allowing for about 10% error, state inactive mine reclamation program staff equate the radon ALARA goal to a PAEC concentration of 0.33 WL (1.55 WLM·y^{-1}), which is used to trigger respiratory protection. If one assumes the NIOSH-preferred DCF (excluding error), then the state inactive mine reclamation program radon goal reduces to 1 5 WLM·y^{-1}. Conversely, applying the 800 hour occupancy to the NIOSH-recommended reference level of 1 WLM·y^{-1} results in a PAEC concentration of 0.2 WL.

CONCLUSIONS

Monitoring results and onsite observations during this HHE suggest that ionizing radiation hazards during mine closure activities are relatively low overall; however, radon exposures necessitating intervention can occur at some work locations. Limiting occupancy, simple engineering controls (i.e , barriers, ventilation), and the use of respiratory protection in some/certain situations are the preferred control measures for keeping radon exposures ALARA. Extreme differences in observed radon concentrations between and within adits suggests that knowledge of environmental factors (moisture, ventilation patterns, weather conditions) and a rigorous monitoring plan are necessary for appropriate hazard characterization. Employers and employees together must remain vigilant in identification, characterization, and mitigation of radon hazards in the workplace through training, monitoring practices, and application of control measures. Low-level gamma radiation fields at the surface of waste rock piles and near mine adits also may contribute to the ionizing radiation hazard; however, on the basis of our observations, intervention is rarely needed and may be limited to the case of reducing exposures to the declared pregnant worker.

RECOMMENDATIONS

On the basis of our findings, we recommend the actions listed below to create a more healthful workplace. Our recommendations are based on the hierarchy of controls approach (Appendix). This approach groups actions by their likely effectiveness in reducing or removing hazards. In most cases, the preferred approach is to eliminate hazardous materials or processes and install engineering controls to reduce exposure or shield employees. Until such controls are in place, or if they are not effective or feasible, administrative measures and/or personal protective equipment may be needed.

This hierarchy can be summarized as follows:
- Elimination
- Substitution
- Engineering controls
- Administrative controls
- Personal protective equipment

Control methods at the top of the list are potentially more effective and protective than those at the bottom. Following the hierarchy normally leads to the implementation of inherently safer systems, ones where the risk of illness or injury has been substantially reduced.

RECOMMENDATIONS (CONTINUED)

Elimination and substitution, while most effective at reducing hazards, also tend to be the most difficult to implement in an existing process and do not apply to radon exposures during the construction of mine closures. Engineering controls, the next tier in the hierarchy, are used to remove a hazard or place a barrier between the employee and the hazard. The use of engineering controls is hampered by the extreme conditions common to the remote mining areas. Permanent electrical power is unusual, and the rugged terrain makes transporting equipment to job sites difficult and potentially hazardous. Nevertheless, simple controls involving portable equipment may offer improvements in risk reduction over administrative controls or respiratory protection.

Administrative controls are management-dictated work practices and policies to reduce or prevent exposures to workplace hazards. The effectiveness of administrative changes in work practices for controlling workplace hazards is dependent on management commitment and employee acceptance. Regular monitoring and reinforcement are necessary to ensure that control policies and procedures are not circumvented in the name of convenience or production.

PPE is the least effective means for controlling employee exposures. Proper use of PPE requires a comprehensive program and calls for a high level of employee involvement and commitment to be effective. The use of PPE requires the choice of the appropriate equipment to reduce the hazard and the development of supporting programs such as training, change-out schedules, and medical assessment if needed. PPE should not be relied upon as the sole method for limiting employee exposures. Rather, PPE should be used until engineering and administrative controls can be demonstrated to be effective in limiting exposures to acceptable levels.

This HHE addresses the hazards associated with ionizing radiation exposure during closure work at the mine entry point, but not within the mine. In selecting controls, specific working conditions at these remote mine sites must be considered. Undue focus on radiological risks at these sites may undermine appropriate consideration of other significant occupational hazards. Other uncharacterized closure activities, such as assessing wildlife habitation of the mine, may require prolonged underground occupancy, which is likely to introduce a different set of occupational hazards and require modification or addition to the controls recommended in this report. Employers are encouraged to use the following recommendations on engineering

RECOMMENDATIONS (CONTINUED)

and administrative controls to minimize potential radiation hazards during closure activities, but should also conduct task-specific job hazard analyses to ensure that ALARA goals are maintained during all work activities. In particular, additional hazard characterization is needed for jobs requiring mine occupancy.

Engineering Controls

1. Construct temporary barriers at mine openings. Our limited evaluation of the barrier at Adit 908A3 suggested that a simple temporary barrier may substantially reduce radiation hazards from mine outcasting. The barrier could be constructed onsite from plastic sheeting and a stick frame. Even a loose fitting barrier should reduce airborne radon concentrations in the immediate area of an outcasting mine opening. The effectiveness of the barrier can be ascertained by confirmatory radon monitoring.

2. Use dilution ventilation when possible, particularly when average radon concentrations are above 1 WL. Directing vent fans toward or across the mine opening may help to offset outcasting. Portable battery-powered fans may be sufficient to lower average radon concentrations to below 0.1 WL. Industrial fans powered by portable gas-powered generators may be required in rare situations where average breathing zone radon concentrations are likely to exceed 1.0 WL.

Administrative Controls

1. Adopt a reference level or ALARA goal for requiring intervention (i.e., engineering, administrative, or PPE controls). For example, a reference level of 10 mSv effective dose from radon progeny in a working year is consistent with the recommendations of the ICRP and existing NIOSH recommendations for radon exposures in uranium miners. This reference level is well below regulatory limits but is readily achievable in occupational settings associated with mine closure activities.

2. Increase sample frequency and/or duration to improve the precision of exposure estimates. If CWLMs are used, then, in addition to lengthening sampling periods, the instruments should be tested and/or calibrated in a radon chamber

over the range of anticipated exposures. Radon monitoring protocols currently used by the state inactive mine reclamation program may not be sufficient to characterize workplace radon concentrations that widely vary with time. Inexpensive passive monitors that are designed for estimating long-term averages may provide a more suitable alternative to CWLMs.

3. Inform employees about the health risk of ionizing radiation exposure in the workplace (Appendix). In this case, the health risk is primarily excesses in lung cancers from radon exposure and, to a lesser extent, lung and other malignancies from exposures to low linear energy transfer radiation. Training should emphasize methods to identify conditions that can increase the hazard (e.g , outcasting mine, presence of standing water), the controls used to keep individual employee exposures ALARA (e.g., work restrictions, engineering controls, respiratory protection), and personal risk concerns such as pregnancy.

4. Ensure that all preparatory work, such as hazards briefing, job training, gathering native rock, staging tools, and mixing mortar, is conducted in a manner that maximizes work efficiency and reduces the duration of work in the immediate vicinity of the mine opening where the dose is greatest. Further dose reduction may be achieved through work restrictions. The employer could restrict the stay time for individuals in the work area to ensure that annual doses remain below the reference level. Given that none of the closure work we observed resulted in occupancies at mine opening approaching a full work shift, simple stay time restrictions may be an effective control measure. As an alternative, stay times could be assigned to individuals rather than to the work group. In most cases, the area of greatest hazard is small and cannot be simultaneously occupied by many employees. Rotating employees through the area during the course of work distributes the collective dose from the job more evenly to all employees thereby reducing the exposure to any single worker. If stay times are used, the employer should keep a record of the times in the area to reconstruct doses at a later time.

5. Appropriately use personal dosimetry. On the basis of the dose measurements by NIOSH and data obtained from the state inactive mine reclamation program, there is little evidence supporting the need for personal dose monitoring. Nonetheless, some employers may issue dosimetry to their

employees as a precaution. If dosimeters are used, the equipment and monitoring cycle should be selected on the basis of the low daily dose expected (i.e., <40 µSv), and employers should keep records of exposures according to applicable standards.

Personal Protective Equipment - Radon

1. Wear NIOSH-approved respirators for radionuclides and radon daughters in situations where barriers, ventilation, and administrative controls are insufficient to ensure that a worker's annual radon exposure will not exceed 1.0 WLM. To ensure proper selection, maintenance, and use of respirators, respiratory protection should be provided in the context of a written respiratory protection program that meets the requirements in the OSHA respiratory protection standard [29 CFR 1910.134]. More information on the OSHA respiratory protection standard is available at http://www.osha.gov/SLTC/respiratoryprotection/index.html.

REFERENCES

CFR. Code of Federal Regulations. Washington, DC: U.S. Government Printing Office, Office of the Federal Register.

Duraski R [2010]. Construction worker radiation exposure at abandoned uranium mines. Bureau of Land Management, New Mexico State Office. Unpublished draft.

ICRP [2007]. The 2007 recommendations of the International Commission on Radiological Protection. ICRP Publication 103. Ann ICRP 37(2-4):1–332.

Kendall GM, Smith TJ [2002]. Doses to organs and tissues from radon and its decay products. J Radiol Prot 22(4):389–406.

Kendall GM, Fell TP, Harrison JD [2009]. Dose to red bone marrow of infants, children and adults from radiation of natural origin. J Radiol Prot 29(2):123–138.

Richardson RB, Eatough JP, Henshaw DL [1991]. Dose to red bone marrow from natural radon and thoron exposure. Br J Radiol 64(763):608–624.

Appendix: Occupational Exposure Limits and Health Effects

In evaluating the hazards posed by workplace exposures, NIOSH investigators use both mandatory (legally enforceable) and recommended OELs for chemical, physical, and biological agents as a guide for making recommendations. OELs have been developed by federal agencies and safety and health organizations to prevent the occurrence of adverse health effects from workplace exposures. Generally, OELs suggest levels of exposure that most employees may be exposed to for up to 10 hours per day, 40 hours per week, for a working lifetime, without experiencing adverse health effects. However, not all employees will be protected from adverse health effects even if their exposures are maintained below these levels.

In the United States, OELs have been established by federal agencies, professional organizations, state and local governments, and other entities. Some OELs are legally enforceable limits, while others are recommendations. The U.S. Department of Labor OSHA PELs (29 CFR 1910 [general industry]; 29 CFR 1926 [construction industry]; and 29 CFR 1917 [maritime industry]) are legal limits enforceable in workplaces covered under the Occupational Safety and Health Act of 1970. NIOSH RELs are recommendations based on a critical review of the scientific and technical information available on a given hazard and the adequacy of methods to identify and control the hazard. NIOSH also recommends different types of risk management practices (e.g., engineering controls, safe work practices, employee education/training, personal protective equipment, and exposure and medical monitoring) to minimize the risk of exposure and adverse health effects from these hazards. Other OELs that are commonly used and cited in the United States include the TLVs recommended by ACGIH, a professional organization. The TLVs are developed by ACGIH committee members from a review of the published, peer-reviewed literature. ACGIH TLVs are not consensus standards. TLVs are considered voluntary exposure guidelines for use by industrial hygienists and others trained in this discipline "to assist in the control of health hazards" [ACGIH 2011].

Employers should understand that not all hazardous chemicals and physical agents have specific OSHA PELs, and for some agents the legally enforceable and recommended limits may not reflect current health-based information. However, an employer is still required by OSHA to protect its employees from hazards even in the absence of a specific OSHA PEL. OSHA requires an employer to furnish employees a place of employment free from recognized hazards that cause or are likely to cause death or serious physical harm [Occupational Safety and Health Act of 1970 (Public Law 91–596, sec. 5(a)(1))]. Thus, NIOSH investigators encourage employers to make use of other OELs and exposure guidelines when making risk assessments and risk management decisions to best protect the health of their employees. NIOSH investigators also encourage the use of the traditional hierarchy of controls approach to eliminate or minimize identified workplace hazards. This includes, in order of preference, the use of (1) substitution or elimination of the hazardous agent, (2) engineering controls (e g., local exhaust ventilation, process enclosure, dilution ventilation), (3) administrative controls (e.g., limiting time of exposure, employee training, work practice changes, medical surveillance), and (4) personal protective equipment (e g , respiratory protection, gloves, eye protection, hearing protection). Control banding, a qualitative risk assessment and risk management tool, is a complementary approach to protecting employee health that focuses resources on exposure controls by describing how a risk needs to be managed. Information on control banding is available at http://www.cdc gov/niosh/topics/ctrlbanding/. This approach can be applied in situations where OELs have not been established or can be used to supplement the OELs, when available.

Below we provide OELs and exposure guidelines for alpha and gamma radiation, as well as a discussion of the potential health effects from exposure to ionizing radiation.

Radon

Radon is a colorless, odorless, inert, radioactive noble gas that has three isotopic forms found ubiquitously in nature: ^{222}Rn, which is a member of the ^{238}U decay chain; ^{220}Rn (commonly known as "thoron"), which is in the decay chain of ^{232}Th; and ^{219}Rn (known as "actinon"), which results from the decay of ^{235}U. Of the three forms, ^{222}Rn and its subsequent radioactive decay products present the greatest risk in most environmental and occupational settings because of its natural abundance. ^{222}Rn undergoes radioactive decays via a series of solid short-lived radionuclides (i.e., polonium-218, lead-214, bismuth-214, and polonium-214), commonly referred to as "radon progeny" or "radon daughters." These decay products appear either as unattached ions or are attached to condensation nuclei or dust particles, forming a respirable radioactive aerosol.

Environmental levels of radon in the United States vary widely, with average indoor concentrations in U.S. homes of about 46 Bq·m^{-3} and in Colorado homes of 96 Bq·m^{-3} [Marcinowski et al. 1994]. Outdoor radon concentrations tend to be much lower with national and regional (Nevada and Colorado) averages of about 15 Bq·m^{-3} [Price et al. 1994; Borak and Baynes 1999], but progeny equilibrium is typically greater outdoors [NCRP 2009]. NCRP estimates that radon progeny exposure accounts for about 36% of the total dose received by the U.S. population annually [NCRP 2009]. The main contributor to tissue absorbed dose is densely ionizing radiation in the form of alpha particles from the decay of respired short-lived radon progeny; therefore, the organ most at risk from exposure is the lung, primarily from deposition of radon progeny in the bronchial epithelium. Dose to other organs and the fetus from inhaled radon progeny are at least an order of magnitude less than that of the lung [Kendall and Smith 2002]. Numerous studies of underground uranium miners who were exposed to relatively high levels of radon have unequivocally established radon as a human lung carcinogen [IARC 1988]. EPA claims that radon is the second leading cause of lung cancer in the United States and is the leading cause among persons who never smoked. The estimated risk from lifetime exposure at the EPA action level of 150 Bq·m^{-3} (4 pCi·L^{-1}) is 2.3% [EPA 2003].

Much less information is available on other health outcomes associated with radon exposure. There is sparse evidence suggesting increased leukemia in uranium miners exposed to radon [Darby et al. 1995; Rericha et al. 2006] although most miner studies have not shown similar results [Tomasek et al. 1993; Laurier et al. 2004; Mohner et al. 2006; Schubauer-Berigan et al. 2009; Lane et al. 2010]. Some researchers have postulated that radon progeny that is deposited on skin surfaces can result in non-negligible dose to sensitive basal cells, which may result in increased incidence of non-melanoma skin cancer [Sevcova et al. 1978; Eatough and Henshaw 1991; Denman et al. 2003]. The current weight of evidence is insufficient to establish a causal link between radon and skin cancer in humans [Charles 2007a; Charles 2007b].

APPENDIX: OCCUPATIONAL EXPOSURE LIMITS AND HEALTH EFFECTS (CONTINUED)

Terminology, Units and Dose

Airborne radioactivity concentrations specific to radon exposures are typically expressed as PAEC, whereby PAEC is the sum of the alpha energy emitted by decay of atoms from any mixture of short-lived radon progeny within a unit volume of air. The quantity is expressed in units of $J \cdot m^{-3}$ where $1 \ J \cdot m^{-3} = 6.242 \times 1012$ $MeV \cdot m^{-3}$. PAEC is often defined in terms of WL where $1 \ WL = 1.3 \times 108 \ MeV \cdot m^{-3}$ ($1.3 \times 105 \ MeV \cdot L^{-1}$). Radon progeny exposure is typically quantified as the time integral of PAEC and is expressed in units of $J \cdot h \cdot m^{-3}$. The historical unit of exposure is the WLM, which is defined as exposure to a PAEC of 1 WL for one month (170 hours); therefore, $1 \ WLM = 3.54 \ mJ \cdot h \cdot m^{-3}$. Exposures have also been quantified in terms of EEC of ^{222}Rn gas, where $1 \ kBq \cdot m^{-3}$ of ^{222}Rn in 100% equilibrium = $5.56 \times 10^{-6} \ J \cdot m^{-3}$ (i.e., $100 \ pCi \cdot L^{-1} = 1$ WL). F_{eq} is the ratio of the EEC to the activity concentration of ^{222}Rn; therefore, a measured radon concentration of $1 \ kBq \cdot m^{-3}$ that is in 40% equilibrium (i.e., $F_{eq} = 0.4$) will give a PAEC of = $2.22 \times 10^{-6} \ J \cdot m^{-3}$ (0.4 WL).

Radiation exposure standards are typically expressed in units of E, which is a radiation protection quantity used to describe "dose" in terms of equivalence to uniform whole-body exposure to low linear energy transfer radiation. Thus, by accounting for various types of radiation and body tissues, the risk from absorbed dose to lung tissue from densely ionizing radiation (e.g., radon PAEC) can be related to the stochastic risk caused by uniform whole body exposures to gamma radiation. By definition:

$$E = \sum_T w_T \sum_R w_R \cdot D_{T,R}$$

where w_R and w_T are the radiation and tissue weighting factors, and $D_{T,R}$ is the mean absorbed dose in tissue or organ T due to incident radiation R. The unit of effective dose is the joule per kilogram and is called the Sv. In the case of radon progeny, the target tissue is the lung ($w_T = 0.12$), and alpha particles are given a radiation weight of 20 under standard ICRP recommendations [ICRP 1992].

The ratio of effective dose to the total exposure to radon progeny is referred to as the DCF. In its Publication 65, ICRP recommended an epidemiologic-based DCF for occupationally exposed individuals of $5 \ mSv \cdot WLM^{-1}$ [ICRP 1993]. This value was obtained by direct comparison of the detriment associated with a unit exposure to radon, as determined by studies of uranium miners, to the detriment associated with a unit effective dose, as determined principally from studies of Japanese atomic bomb survivors. The ICRP [ICRP 2009; ICRP 2010] has recently reexamined the results from epidemiological studies of miners and now recommends a lifetime excess absolute risk of 5×10^{-4} per WLM (14×10^{-5} per $mJ \cdot h \cdot m^{-3}$) for radon and radon progeny induced lung cancer, compared to the previous value of 2.8×10^{-4} per WLM (8×10^{-5} per $mJ \cdot h \cdot m^{-3}$). This change in the detriment suggests a concomitant two-fold increase to the DCF value (i.e., $10 \ mSv \cdot WLM^{-1}$).

Dosimetric-based DCFs for radon are widely available in the literature as a substitute for the risk-based approach [Stather 2004; Kranrod et al. 2010; Hofmann and Winkler-Heil 2011]. DCF values vary from differences in modeling assumptions, such as breathing rate, unattached fraction, and weighting factors for tissues and radiation quality (Table A1). (See Table A2 for radon terms and unit conversions.) Most DCFs from reference biokinetic and dosimetric models report a higher dose per unit exposure than that found in ICRP Publication 65 and appear more in line with recent ICRP findings on radon-induced lung cancer risk. In 2009, the ICRP acknowledged these differences and stated that revisions to the recommended DCF are likely to increase the estimate of the effective dose per unit exposure by twofold [ICRP 2009; ICRP 2010]. Given these findings, we used a DCF value of 10 mSv·WLM^{-1} in subsequent calculations in this report.

Table A1. Various radon dose conversion factors (DCFs)

Source	Model basis	Exposure place	DCF (mSv·WLM^{-1})
[ICRP 1993]	epidemiologic	workplaces	5
[ICRP 1981]	dosimetric	indoors and outdoors	10
[NCRP 2009]	dosimetric	indoors and outdoors	10
[UNSCEAR 2008]*	dosimetric	indoors and outdoors	5.7
[Winkler-Heil et al. 2007]	dosimetric	mines	8.3–11.8, avg. ~9
[Nikezic et al. 2006]	dosimetric	NS†	14.2
[Porstendörfer and Reineking 1999]	dosimetric	workplaces	5.7–13
[Kranrod et al. 2010]	dosimetric	workplaces	10.8
[Marsh et al. 2008]‡	dosimetric	mines	10.8–30.2
[Marsh et al. 2010]	epidemiologic	workplaces	12 based on lifetime detriment 5 based on lung detriment

*UNSCEAR=United Nations Scientific Committee on the Effects of Atomic Radiation
†NS=not specified
‡Assumes w_R=20 and w_T=0.12

There are some instances in which radon measurements are restricted to radon gas, in which case a progeny equilibrium factor is assumed. The degree of disequilibrium is a function of the "age" of the air, progeny deposition (plate-out), and ventilation patterns. Therefore, F_{eq} can vary widely and is likely to be lowest at the adit brow where progeny diffuses into fresh air and highest deep within the abandoned mine where there is little or no ventilation [Gillmore et al. 2011]. Typical values for F_{eq} are 0.4 for indoor air and 0.7 for outdoors [ICRP 1993]. Some studies have suggested that values of F_{eq} in air in and around abandoned mines and caves range between 0.04 and 0.7, with a mean of about 0.4 [Butterwreck et al. 1992; Cavallo 2000; Gillmore et al. 2001; Denman et al. 2003; Gillmore et al. 2011]. A one-hour exposure to a radon gas concentration of 1 kBq·m^{-3} (~ 27 pCi·L^{-1}) at an equilibrium factor, F_{eq}, of 0.4 corresponds to an effective dose of 6.4 μSv; therefore, continuous exposure in a 2,000-hour working year at this level results in approximately 12.8 mSv.

Table A2. Radon terms and unit conversions

Metric	Description	Historic units	SI units	Unit conversions
Activity	Radioactive decay events per unit time	Ci	Bq	1 Ci = 3.7 x 10^{10} Bq
Concentration	Radon gas concentration	pCi·L^{-1}	Bq·m^{-3}	1 pCi·L^{-1} = 37 Bq·m^{-3}
	PAEC	WL	J·m^{-3}	1 WL = 2.08 x 10^{-5} J·m^{-3}
	EEC	pCi·L^{-1}	Bq·m^{-3}	1 Bq·m^{-3} = 5.56 x10^{-9} J·m^{-3} 100 pCi·L^{-1} = 1 WL
Equilibrium factor, F_{eq}	Fraction of potential alpha energy of the short-lived radon progeny, compared to secular equilibrium	NA*	NA	F_{eq} = (0.106 c_{Po-218} + 0.514 c_{Pb-214} + 0.380 c_{Bi-214}) / c_{Rn-222} where c_x stands for the activity concentration of the nuclide x
Exposure	Exposure	WLM	J·h·m^{-3}	1 WLM = 3.54 J·h·m^{-3} 1 WLM = 170 WL·h 1 WLM = 800 Bq·m^{-3} for 2,000 hour occupancy and F_{eq}=0.4
Dose	D†	rad‡	Gy	100 rad = 1 Gy
	E§	rem¶	Sv	100 rem = 1 Sv

*NA=not applicable
†*D*=Absorbed dose
‡rad=radiation absorbed dose
§*E*=Effective dose or weighted equivalent dose
¶rem=roentgen equivalent man

Gamma and X-rays

External Dose

Gamma rays are penetrating high-energy, short-wavelength electromagnetic radiation emitted from the nucleus of an atom undergoing radioactive decay. X-rays are electromagnetic radiation originating outside of the nucleus; therefore, they are indistinguishable from gamma-rays and differ only by their origin. Both gamma and x-rays are a form of ionizing radiation, which is known to cause cancers in most tissues, in most species, and in all ages including the fetus [Little 2000].

Gamma and x-ray radiation exposure is ubiquitous and results from both terrestrial and cosmic sources. The NCRP estimates that the average U.S. adult male receives 0 56 mSv annually from external irradiation by ubiquitous background sources; 0.21 mSv from terrestrial sources; and 0.33 from cosmic radiation [NCRP 2009]. Average absorbed dose rates from terrestrial sources in the United States range from <6 $nGy\cdot h^{-1}$ to >83 $nGy\cdot h^{-1}$ [Duval et al. 2005]. Cosmic-ray dose rates are slightly higher, ranging from <40 $nGy\cdot h^{-1}$ to >88 $nGy\cdot h^{-1}$ [Duval et al. 2005]. Western states tend to have higher dose rates due to increased amounts of naturally occurring radioactive material and increased elevation. Typical absorbed dose rates in the Four Corner region range from 0.1 $\mu Gy\cdot h^{-1}$ to 0.4 $\mu Gy\cdot h^{-1}$ [EPA 2008]. Elevated gamma radiation is likely in areas around overburden, subeconomic ore (protore), or waste rock piles in which increased levels of radium are present. The radium content is roughly proportional to the uranium content in raw materials. Dose rate measurements (including background) taken by the EPA at overburden piles in U.S. mining sites typically ranged from 0.2 $\mu Sv\cdot h^{-1}$ to 3.0 $\mu Sv\cdot h^{-1}$ with an average value of 0.5 $\mu Sv\cdot h^{-1}$. Dose rates at protore piles were higher, with an average value of 3.5 $\mu Sv\cdot h^{-1}$ and a range of 0.8 $\mu Sv\cdot h^{-1}$ to 12.5 $\mu Sv\cdot h^{-1}$ [EPA 2008].

Occupational Exposure Limits

NIOSH-Recommended Exposure Limit

In October 1987, NIOSH published its recommended standard for occupational exposure to radon progeny in underground mines [NIOSH 1987]. The primary goal of these recommendations was to decrease the risk of lung cancer in underground uranium miners over a working lifetime of 30 years. Exposure limits were derived from (1) risk models that used information on protracted radon exposures in the mining industry, (2) values that were measureable and reproducible, and (3) limits that could be achieved with available technology. NIOSH made several recommendations in this publication, including:

- *"Exposure to radon progeny in underground mines shall not exceed 1 WLM per year, and the average work shift concentration shall not exceed 1/12 of 1 WL (or 0.083 WL). The REL of 1 WLM per year is an upper limit of exposure, and every effort shall be made to reduce exposures to the lowest levels possible..."* [Section 2(a)].

- *"Grab samples for radon progeny in the workplace shall be taken and analyzed using working level monitors, the Kusnetz method, or any other method at least equivalent in accuracy, precision, and sensitivity."* [Section 2(b)].

- *"All operators of underground mines shall perform environmental evaluations in all work areas to determine exposures to radon progeny...If environmental monitoring in a work area indicates that the average work shift concentration of radon progeny exceeds 1/12 WL, the mine operator shall prepare an action plan describing the types of engineering controls and work practices that will be implemented to reduce the average work shift concentration in that area."* [Section 3(a) (1) and (3)].

Appendix: Occupational Exposure Limits and Health Effects (continued)

- *"The mine operator shall institute a medical surveillance program for all miners." [Section 4(a) (1)].*

- *"Respiratory protection shall be used by miners (1) when work practices and engineering controls are not adequate to limit average work shift concentrations of radon progeny to 1/12 WL, (2) when entering a mine area where concentrations or radon progeny are unknown, or (3) during emergencies ..." [Section 7(a)].*

The NIOSH REL of 1 WLM·y^{-1} results in an annual effective dose that is fivefold less than current U.S. occupational standards for whole-body irradiation [10 CFR 835, Appendix C; 10 CFR 20, Appendix B, Table 1; 29 CFR 1910.1096; 29 CFR 1926.53] and one half of that observed in most international settings (i.e., 20 mSv·y^{-1}, averaged over 5 years, as recommended by the ICRP [ICRP 1992].

OSHA Standards for General Industry and Construction

OSHA established a PEL for radon at 3.7 kBq·m^{-3} (100 pCi·L^{-1}) averaged over a work week, which results in a cumulative exposure in a working year (2,000 hours) of 12 WLM, assuming 100% progeny equilibrium [29 CFR 1910.1096; 29 CFR 1926 53]. The OSHA PEL was based on the now obsolete values from the 1969 revision of 10 CFR 20, which relied on the earlier recommendations by the Federal Radiation Council of 12 WLM·y^{-1}. Nevertheless, OSHA also requires employers to limit doses to 12.5 mSv in a calendar quarter [29 CFR 1910.1096 (b)(1)]; therefore, an effective radon control limit of 5 WLM per year is inferred, provided "dose" includes the effective dose from radon, and the DCF is 10 mSv·WLM^{-1}.

Whole Body Dose

For those 18 years old or older, OSHA states that persons working in a "restricted area" shall be limited to doses to the whole body (head and trunk, active blood-forming organs, lens of eyes, or gonads) to no more than 12.5 mSv in any period of one calendar quarter [29 CFR 1910.1096]. A restricted area is defined as any area where access is controlled by the employer for purposes of protection of individuals from exposure to radiation or radioactive materials [29 CFR 1910.1096(a)(3)]. OSHA allows this limit to be exceeded provided that the dose does not exceed 30 mSv in any calendar quarter [29 CFR 1910.1096(b)(2)(i)]; the lifetime occupational dose remains below 5(N−18), where N is the age of the worker [29 CFR 1910.1096(b)(2)(ii)]; and the employer maintains adequate exposure records to show that these conditions have not been violated) [29 CFR 1910.1096(b)(2)(iii)]. On the basis of these constraints and using the DCF of 10 mSv·WLM^{-1}, one may derive an applicable exposure standard of 1.25 WLM in any calendar quarter or a continuous average exposure in a work shift of no more than about 0.4 WL.

Airborne Radioactivity

In regard to airborne radioactivity standards, OSHA currently sets the maximum permissible concentration for ^{222}Rn at 3.7 kBq·m^{-3} (100 pCi·L^{-1}) for 40 hours in any work week of 7 consecutive days [29 CFR 1910.1096(c)(1)]. Thus, assuming an equilibrium fraction of 100%, continuous workplace exposures at the maximum permissible concentration (1 WL) result in 3.0 WLM per quarter.

Appendix: Occupational Exposure Limits and Health Effects (Continued)

Personal Monitoring

OSHA requires personal monitoring of adult employees who enter a restricted area and are likely to receive a dose in any calendar quarter that exceeds 3.125 mSv [29 CFR 1910.1096(d)(2)(i)].

Other Recommendations and Standards

The NIOSH REL was intended for the protection of underground uranium miners and was meant for consideration in regulations promulgated by MSHA. Nevertheless, MSHA has not revised its annual exposure limit of 4 WLM [40 CFR 57 5038], which was initially adopted for U.S. miners in 1971. The current MSHA limit has also been embraced by the NRC, which specifies an ALI for occupational exposures of 4 WLM [10 CFR 20, Appendix B, Table 1]. The U.S. annual limit of 4 WLM was initially selected by the Federal Radiation Council on the basis of the feasibility of managing exposures in the uranium mining industry. However, subsequent dosimetric and epidemiologic-based models in ICRP Publication 32 [ICRP 1981] concluded that the DCF for radon progeny was ~ 10 mSv·WLM^{-1}. That is, the effective dose from 4 WLM exposures was approximately equal to the regulatory dose limits in place at that time.

Not all U.S. regulating agencies limit annual occupational radon exposures to 4 WLM. DOE uses an ALI of 10 WLM, which is based on the ICRP recommendations of a dose conversion convention of 5 mSv·WLM^{-1} [ICRP 1993].

In large part, countries outside of the United States have adopted the most recent recommendations of the ICRP [ICRP 1993], whereby occupational radon exposures are summed with other sources of radiation, and the total dose is limited to 20 mSv·y^{-1} averaged over 5 years and less than 50 mSv in any one year (Table A3).

In this context, the DCF is assumed to be 5 mSv·WLM^{-1}; therefore, the equivalent annual radon exposure limit is 14 mJ·h·m^{-3} (4 WLM) averaged over 5 years, not to exceed 35 mJ·h·m^{-3} (10 WLM) in any one year.

Table A3. Occupational radon regulations, guidance, and recommended limits

Agency	Regulation / Recommendation	Covered Facilities	Radon Limits	Total Exposure Limit	Intervention, Reference or Control levels
ICRP [ICRP 2011]	Publication No. 115	Domestic and occupational exposure	Lifetime lung cancer EAR*=5 × 10^{-4} per WLM		
ICRP [ICRP 2007]	Publication No. 103	Domestic and occupational exposure	Applicable limits consistent with ICRP Publication 65	Applicable limits consistent with ICRP Publication 60	<10 mSv·y^{-1} (<1.5 kBq·m^{-3})
ICRP [ICRP 1992; ICRP 1993]	Publication No. 65 (radon) Publication No. 60 (total dose)	Domestic and occupational exposure	Lifetime lung cancer EAR=2.8 × 10^{-4} per WLM 14 mJ·h·m^{-3} (20 mSv; 4 WLM, 3 kBq·m^{-3}) 35 mJ·h·m^{-3} (50 mSv; 10 WLM, 8 kBq·m^{-3})	< 20 mSv·y^{-1} averaged over 5 years, not to exceed 50 mSv in any year	3–10 mSv·y^{-1} (0.5–1.5 kBq·m^{-3}) 1 kBq·m^{-3}=6 mSv based on 2,000 hour occupancy, F_{eq} =0.4
NCRP [NCRP 1984]	Report No. 77	Domestic and occupational exposure	Lifetime lung cancer EAR=1.5 × 10^{-4} per WLM 2 WLM·y^{-1}	5 mSv·y^{-1} in areas of enhanced levels of the uranium series. Not additive; radon considered to be controlling	
ACGIH [ACGIH 2011]	2011 TLVs® and BEIs®		TLV=4 WLM·y^{-1}	Limits consistent with ICRP Publication 60	
NIOSH [NIOSH 1987]	Publication No. 88-101	Underground mines	REL=1 WLM·y^{-1}	Not addressed	1/12 WL (0.083 WL) per working shift
IAEA† [IAIA 2003]	Basic Safety Standard 115 and Safety Report Series No. 33	All workplaces (includes exposure to naturally occurring radon not related to production activities)	Limits consistent with ICRP Publication 65	Limits consistent with ICRP Publication 60	Potential remediation measures discussed
IAEA [IAEA 2004]	Safety Guide No. RS-G-1.6	Activities involved in the mining and processing of raw materials	Limits consistent with ICRP Publication 65	Limits consistent with ICRP Publication 60	Respirators recommended only for short duration tasks

Table A3. Occupational radon regulations, guidance, and recommended limits (continued)

Agency	Regulation / Recommendation	Covered Facilities	Radon Limits	Total Exposure Limit	Intervention, Reference or Control levels
MSHA [CFR]	30 CFR Part 57 57.5038	Underground mines	4 WLM·y^{-1}	Not addressed	Respiratory protection required at levels ≥1 WL. Air-supplied respiratory protection required at levels ≥10 WL
NRC [CFR]	10 CFR 20, Appendix B, Table 1	NRC Licensees	ALI=4 WLM (14 mJ·h·m^{-3}) , gas (without progeny) 1 mCi (37 MBq) DAC‡: Progeny, 0.33 WL (EEC=30 pCi·L^{-1}); radon gas (without progeny) 148 kBq·m^{-3} (4,000 pCi·L^{-1})	Total Effective Dose Equivalent of 50 mSv (5 rem)	Posting and control at 0.6 ALI, 12-DAC·h (0.1 WL continuous) averaged over one work week Individual monitoring required for adults likely to receive 0.4 WLM in one year
OSHA [CFR]	29 CFR 1910.1096 29 CFR 1926.53	Those not regulated by the U.S. Atomic Energy Act of 1954.	100 pCi·L^{-1} (~3.7 kBq·m^{-3}) 12 WLM·y^{-1} EEC	Combining internal and external sources is not directly addressed; however, "dose" is limited to <12.5 mSv in any calendar quarter.	Posting and control at 25% of the exposure limit averaged over one work week, 25 pCi·L^{-1} (~1 kBq·m^{-3}) in occupied areas
DOE [CFR]	10 CFR 835, Appendix A	DOE facilities	DAC EEC=3 kBq·m^{-3} (80 pCi·L^{-1}); 0.83 WL ALI=10 WLM	Total Effective Dose Equivalent of 50 mSv (5 rem)	Posting and control at 12-DAC·h (0.25 WL continuous) in one work week (0.06 WLM). Air monitoring required for individual likely to receive an exposure of 40 or more DAC-hours (0.2 WLM) in a year Individual monitoring required for adults likely to receive a committed effective dose of 1 mSv (0.2 WLM) in one year

Table A3. Occupational radon regulations, guidance, and recommended limits (continued)

Agency	Regulation / Recommendation	Covered Facilities	Radon Limits	Total Exposure Limit	Intervention, Reference or Control levels
ARPANSA§ [ARPANSA 2005]	Radiation Protection Series Publication No. 9	Australian facilities	Limits consistent with ICRP Publication 65	Limits consistent with ICRP Publication 60	Radiation protection is required if long-term ^{222}Rn >1 kBq·m^{-3}
CNSC¶ [CNSC 2000]	SOR/2000-203	Canadian nuclear facilities	Limits consistent with ICRP Publication 65	Limits consistent with ICRP Publication 60	
HSE** [HSE 1999]	Ionising radiations regulations 1999 No. 3232	UK†† nuclear facilities	Limits consistent with ICRP Publication 65	Limits consistent with ICRP Publication 60	^{222}Rn gas concentration in air, averaged over 24-hour period >400 Bq·m^{-3} (11 pCi·L^{-1}) ^{222}Rn progeny in air averaged over 8-hour period > 6.24×10^{-7} J·m^{-3} (0.03 WL)

*EAR: Excess absolute risk
†IAEA: International Atomic Energy Agency
‡DAC: Derived air concentration
§ARPANSA: Australian Radiation Protection and Nuclear Safety Agency
¶CNSC: Canadian Nuclear Safety Commission
**HSE: United Kingdom (UK) Health and Safety Executive
††UK: United Kingdom

Appendix: Occupational Exposure Limits and Health Effects (continued)

References

ACGIH [2011]. 2011 TLVs® and BEIs®: threshold limit values for chemical substances and physical agents and biological exposure indices. Cincinnati, OH: American Conference of Governmental Industrial Hygienists.

ARPANSA [2005]. Radiation protection and radioactive waste management in mining and mineral processing. Yallambie, Victoria: Australian Radiation Protection and Nuclear Safety Agency, pp. 1–63.

Borak TB, Baynes SA [1999]. Continuous measurements of outdoor ^{222}Rn concentrations for three years at one location in Colorado. Health Phys 76(4):418–420.

Butterwreck G, Porstendörfer J, Reineking A, Kesten J [1992]. Unattached fraction and the aerosol size distribution of the radon progeny in a natural cave and mine atmospheres. Radiat Prot Dosimetry 45(1-4):167–170.

Cavallo AJ [2000]. Understanding mine aerosols for radon risk assessment. J Environ Radioactivity 51(1):99–119.

CFR. Code of Federal Regulations. Washington, D.C., U.S. Government Printing Office, Office of the Federal Register.

Charles MW [2007a]. Radon exposure of the skin: I. Biological effects. J Radiol Prot 27(3):231–252.

Charles MW [2007b]. Radon exposure of the skin: II. Estimation of the attributable risk for skin cancer incidence. J Radiol Prot 27(3):253–274.

CNSC [2000]. Radiation protection regulations. Ottawa, Ontario: Canadian Nuclear Safety Commission, pp. 1–22.

Darby SC, Whitley E, Howe GR, Hutchings SJ, Kusiak RA, Lubin JH, Morrison HI, Tirmarche M, Tomasek L, Radford EP, Roscoe RJ, Samet JM, Yao SH [1995]. Radon and cancers other than lung cancer in underground miners: a collaborative analysis of 11 studies. J Natl Cancer Inst 87(5):378–384.

Denman AR, Eatough JP, Gillmore G, Phillips PS [2003]. Assessment of health risks to skin and lung of elevated radon levels in abandoned mines. Health Phys 85(6):733–739.

Duval JS, Carson JM, Holman PB, Darnley AG [2005]. Terrestrial radioactivity and gamma-ray exposure in the United States and Canada: U.S. Geological Survey Open-File Report 2005-1413. Available online only. Reston, VA: U.S. Geological Survey.

Eatough JP, Henshaw DL [1991]. Radon dose to the skin and the possible induction of skin cancers. Radiat Prot Dosimetry 39(1-3):33–37.

EPA [2003]. EPA assessment of risks from radon in homes. Washington, DC: U.S. Environmental Protection Agency, EPA-402-R-03-003, pp. 1–98.

EPA [2008]. Technical report on technologically enhanced naturally occurring radioactive materials from uranium mining. Volume 1: mining and reclamation background. Washington, DC: U.S. Environmental Protection Agency, EPA 402-R-08-005, pp. 1–225.

Gillmore G, Gharib HA, Denman A, Phillips P, Bridge D [2011]. Radon concentrations in abandoned mines, Cumbria, UK: safety implications for industrial archaeologists. Nat Hazards Earth Syst Sci *11*(5):1311–1318.

Gillmore GK, Phillips P, Denman A, Sperrin M, Pearce G [2001]. Radon levels in abandoned metalliferous mines, Devon, southwest England. Ecotoxicol Environ Saf *49*(3):281–292.

Hofmann W, Winkler-Heil R [2011]. Radon lung dosimetry models. Radiat Prot Dosimetry *145*(2-3):206–212.

HSE [1999]. The ionising radiations regulations 1999. London, United Kingdom: Health and Safety Executive Statutory Instrument 1999 No. 3232, pp. 1–68.

IAEA [2003]. Radiation protection against radon in workplaces other than mines. Vienna, Austria: International Atomic Energy Agency, Safety Reports Series No. 33, pp. 1–79.

IAEA [2004]. Occupational radiation protection in the mining and processing of raw materials. Vienna, Austria: International Atomic Energy Agency, pp. 1–95.

IARC [1988]. Man-made mineral fibres and radon. Vol. 43. Lyon, France: World Health Organization, International Agency for Research on Cancer, pp. 1–300.

ICRP [1981]. Limits for inhalation of radon daughters by workers. ICRP Publication 32. Ann ICRP *6*(1):1–24.

ICRP [1992]. 1990 Recommendations of the International Commission on Radiological Protection. ICRP publication 60. Ann ICRP *21*(1-3):1–201.

ICRP [1993]. Protection against radon-222 at home and at work. ICRP publication 65. Ann ICRP *23*(2):1–45.

ICRP [2007]. The 2007 Recommendations of the International Commission on Radiological Protection. ICRP Publication 103. Ann ICRP *37*(2-4):1–332.

ICRP [2009]. Statement on radon: International Commission on Radiological Protection, ICRP Ref 00/902/09, pp. 1-2.

ICRP [2010]. Lung cancer risk from radon and progeny and statement on radon. ICRP Publication 115. Ann. ICRP 40(1).

Kendall GM, Smith TJ [2002]. Doses to organs and tissues from radon and its decay products. J Radiol Prot 22(4):389–406.

Kranrod C, Ishikawa T, Tokonami S, Sorimachi A, Chanyotha S, Chankow N [2010]. Comparative dosimetry of radon and thoron. Radiat Prot Dosimetry 141(4):424–427.

Lane RS, Frost SE, Howe GR, Zablotska LB [2010]. Mortality (1950–1999) and cancer incidence (1969–1999) in the cohort of Eldorado uranium workers. Radiat Res 174(6):773–785.

Laurier D, Tirmarche M, Mitton N, Valenty M, Richard P, Poveda S, Gelas JM, Quesne B [2004]. An update of cancer mortality among the French cohort of uranium miners: extended follow-up and new source of data for causes of death. Eur J Epidemiol 19(2):139–146.

Little JB [2000]. Radiation carcinogenesis. Carcinogenesis 21(3):397–404.

Marcinowski F, Lucas RM, Yeager WM [1994]. National and regional distributions of airborne radon concentrations in U.S. homes. Health Phys 66(6):699–706.

Marsh JW, Bessa Y, Birchall A, Blanchardon E, Hofmann W, Nosske D, Tomasek L [2008]. Dosimetric models used in the Alpha-Risk project to quantify exposure of uranium miners to radon gas and its progeny. Radiat Prot Dosimetry 130(1):101–106.

Marsh JW, Harrison JD, Laurier D, Blanchardon E, Paquet F, Tirmarche M [2010]. Dose conversion factors for radon: recent developments. Health Phys 99(4):511–516.

Mohner M, Lindtner M, Otten H, Gille HG [2006]. Leukemia and exposure to ionizing radiation among German uranium miners. Am J Ind Med 49(4):238–248.

NCRP [1984]. Exposures from the uranium series with emphasis on radon and its daughters: recommendations of the National Council on Radiation Protection and Measurements. Bethesda, MD: National Council on Radiation Protection and Measurements, Report No. 77, pp. 1–134.

NCRP [2009]. Ionizing radiation exposure of the population of the United States. Bethesda, MD: National Council on Radiation Protection and Measurements, Report No. 160, pp. 1–387.

Nikezic D, Lau BM, Yu KN [2006]. Comparison of dose conversion factors for radon progeny from the ICRP 66 regional model and an airway tube model of tracheo-bronchial tree. Radiat Environ Biophys 45(2):153–157.

NIOSH [1987]. A recommended standard for occupational exposure to radon progeny in underground mines. Washington, DC: U.S. Department of Health and Human Services, Centers for Disease Control, National Institute for Occupational Safety and Health, DHHS (NIOSH) Publication No. 88-101, pp. 1–215.

Porstendorfer J, Reineking A [1999]. Radon: characteristics in air and dose conversion factors. Health Phys 76(3):300–305.

APPENDIX: OCCUPATIONAL EXPOSURE LIMITS AND HEALTH EFFECTS (CONTINUED)

Price JG, Rigby JG, Christensen L, Hess R, LaPointe DD, Ramelli AR, Desilets M, Hopper RD, Kluesner T, Marshall S [1994]. Radon in outdoor air in Nevada. Health Phys 66(4):433–438.

Rericha V, Kulich M, Rericha R, Shore DL, Sandler DP [2006]. Incidence of leukemia, lymphoma, and multiple myeloma in Czech uranium miners: a case-cohort study. Environ Health Perspect 114(6):818–822.

Schubauer-Berigan MK, Daniels RD, Pinkerton LE [2009]. Radon exposure and mortality among white and American Indian uranium miners: an update of the Colorado Plateau cohort. Am J Epidemiol 169(6):718–730.

Sevcova M, Sevc J, Thomas J [1978]. Alpha irradiation of the skin and the possibility of late effects. Health Phys 35(6):803–806.

Stather JW [2004]. Dosimetric and epidemiological approaches to assessing radon doses—can the differences be reconciled? Radiat Prot Dosimetry 112(4):487–492.

Tomasek L, Darby SC, Swerdlow AJ, Placek V, Kunz E [1993]. Radon exposure and cancers other than lung-cancer among uranium miners in west-Bohemia. Lancet 341(8850):919–923.

UNSCEAR [2008]. UNSCEAR 2006 report, vol. II, effects of ionizing radiation. Annex E: sources-to-effects assessment for radon in homes and workplaces. New York: United Nations Scientific Committee on the Effects of Atomic Radiation, pp. 138.

Winkler-Heil R, Hofmann W, Marsh J, Birchall A [2007]. Comparison of radon lung dosimetry models for the estimation of dose uncertainties. Radiat Prot Dosimetry 127(1-4):27–30.

ACKNOWLEDGMENTS AND AVAILABILITY OF REPORT

The Hazard Evaluations and Technical Assistance Branch (HETAB) of the National Institute for Occupational Safety and Health (NIOSH) conducts field investigations of possible health hazards in the workplace. These investigations are conducted under the authority of Section 20(a)(6) of the Occupational Safety and Health Act of 1970, 29 U.S.C. 669(a)(6) which authorizes the Secretary of Health and Human Services, following a written request from any employer or authorized representative of employees, to determine whether any substance normally found in the place of employment has potentially toxic effects in such concentrations as used or found. HETAB also provides, upon request, technical and consultative assistance to federal, state, and local agencies; labor; industry; and other groups or individuals to control occupational health hazards and to prevent related trauma and disease.

Mention of any company or product does not constitute endorsement by NIOSH. In addition, citations to websites external to NIOSH do not constitute NIOSH endorsement of the sponsoring organizations or their programs or products. Furthermore, NIOSH is not responsible for the content of these websites. All Web addresses referenced in this document were accessible as of the publication date.

This report was prepared by Robert D. Daniels of the Occupational Energy Research Program, Industrywide Studies Branch, and David C. Sylvain of HETAB, Division of Surveillance, Hazard Evaluations and Field Studies. Industrial hygiene field assistance was provided by Tim Radtke of the Office of Occupational Safety and Health, U.S. Department of the Interior. Industrial hygiene equipment and logistical support were provided by Donald Booher and Karl Feldmann. Health communication assistance was provided by Stefanie Evans. Editorial assistance was provided by Ellen Galloway. Desktop publishing was performed by Greg Hartle and Mary Winfree.

Copies of this report have been sent to representatives at the federal agency, the state inactive mine reclamation program, the state health department, and the Occupational Safety and Health Administration Regional Office. This report is not copyrighted and may be freely reproduced. The report may be viewed and printed at http://www.cdc.gov/niosh/hhe/. Copies may be purchased from the National Technical Information Service at 5825 Port Royal Road, Springfield, Virginia 22161.